Grief Therapy
for Men

D0921791

Grief Therapy for Men

written by
Linus Mundy

illustrated by
R.W. Alley

ONE
CARING
PLACE

Abbey Press

Text © 1997 by Linus Mundy
Illustrations © 1997 by St. Meinrad Archabbey
Published by One Caring Place
Abbey Press
St. Meinrad, Indiana 47577

Library of Congress Catalog Number
97-77160

ISBN 0-87029-306-0

Printed in the United States of America

Foreword

There are but a few men who know how to grieve well (and the author does not pretend to be one of them). What passes for healthy male grieving in our society usually seems to take the guise of "being strong" and "keeping a stiff upper lip." Worse, men often see it as their role to act bravely so that others—particularly women and children—can do their grieving.

But men—real men—need to grieve, too. Study after study shows males bottling up and burying their sadness deep down where no one can ever see it, only to have it emerge later in body-and-spirit-damaging ways.

Grief Therapy for Men encourages readers not to bury their grief but to bear it and bare it—safely and securely, but openly and honestly. Indeed, there are genuinely masculine ways to grieve well and let true healing happen. You'll find thirty-eight of them inside: practical, specific, and constructive ways to grieve—and grow—as a man.

1.

If you've lost someone you care about, you've earned your "Grieving Permit," no matter how big and strong you are. Some constructive griefwork is now in order.

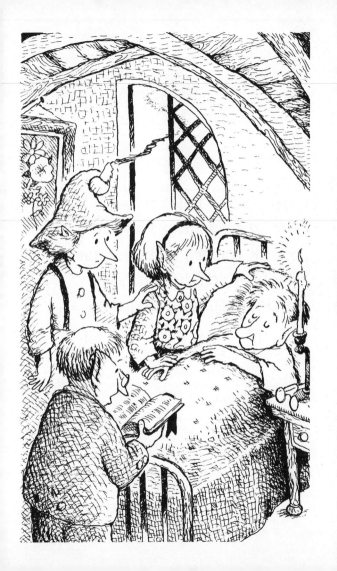

2.

Griefwork is not a waste of time. It's essential for healing parts of yourself you may not even know are broken. Take the time you need to grieve.

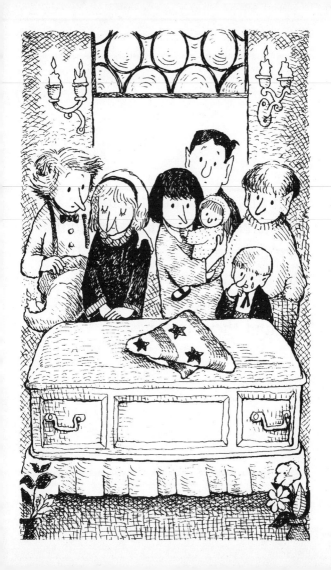

3.

Men are taught always to rise up bravely from a fall—without even dusting themselves off. It's OK to stay down for a little while at least, to compose yourself, and then rise up.

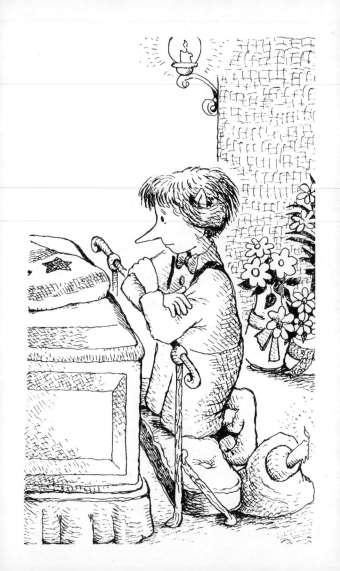

4.

You may be tempted to take the "manly," chin-up approach to grieving. Don't. You'd be cheating an entire side of your humanity and the soul that makes you <u>you</u>.

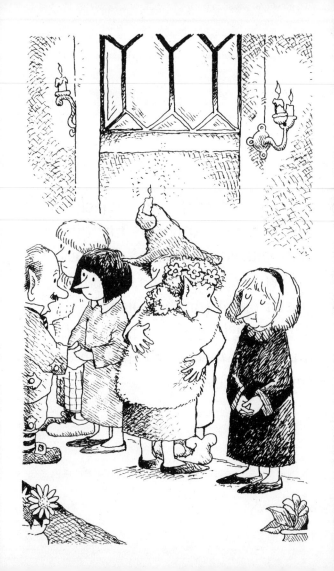

5.

For some men, giving yourself permission to grieve is like giving yourself permission to like flowers or bright colors or dancing or opera (or soap opera). The truth is...grief is universal, and gentle men prefer healing through grieving.

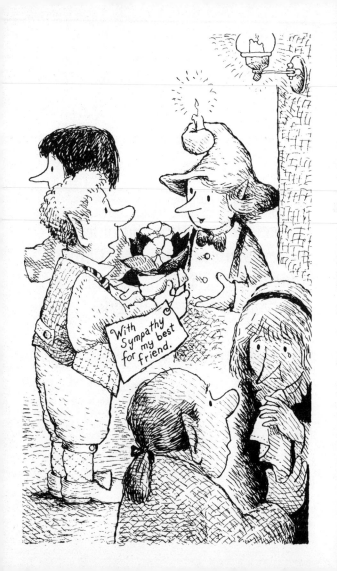

6.

It's good to be a man—to appreciate structure and order, achievement and success. Draw from this reservoir of strength to help you do your griefwork.

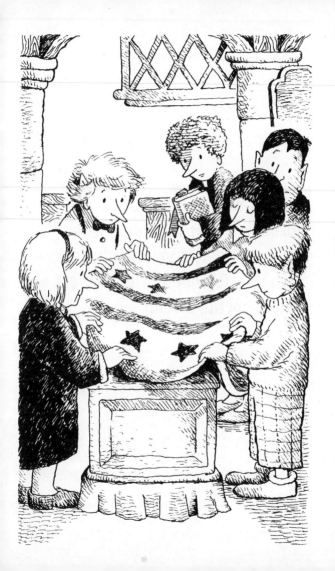

7.

It takes real courage for a real man to get real humble— and human. Let yourself be "weak"—it's one of the greatest ways of being strong.

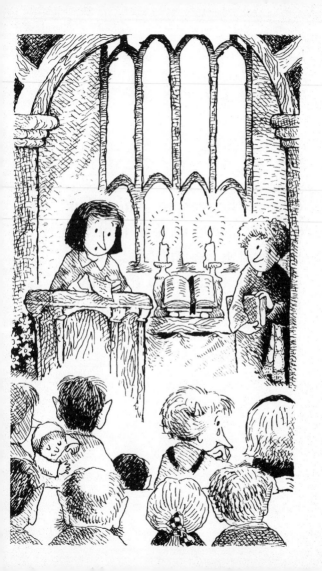

8.

One of the reasons males don't always grieve well is that they may not have had healthy grieving modeled to them by their own fathers. You can change that with your children. Begin now.

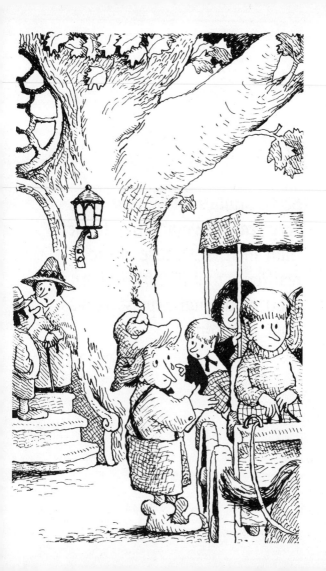

9.

Some studies show that the very reason women live longer than men is because of the resilience and flexibility born of their emotional expressiveness. Take a lesson.

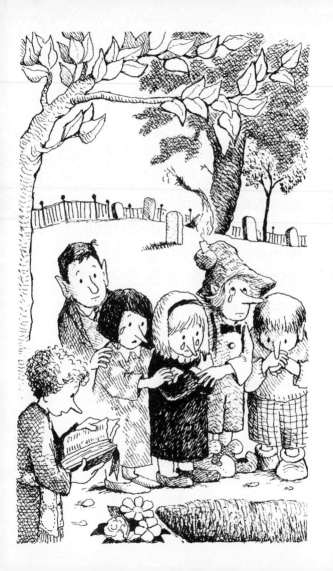

10.

Men tend to hide pain not only from others—but from themselves. This can lead to serious illnesses and disorders. When a man lives in pretense, sooner or later his entire body revolts. Try to find practical, safe ways to reveal your aching heart, little by little.

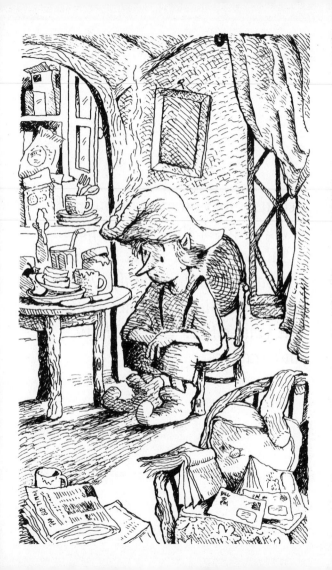

11.

Because men often are ashamed to show grief, they may suffer in silence. If you think grieving and sadness are unmanly, you're not alone. But you're not right. Tell yourself it's OK to show your sadness.

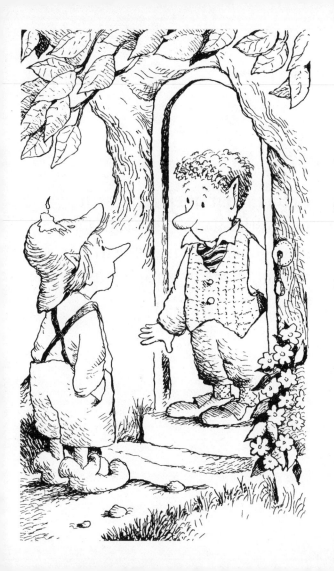

12.

Get out your grief. Express it in healthy ways that work for you—loud or quiet, physical or mental, alone or with a trusted friend.

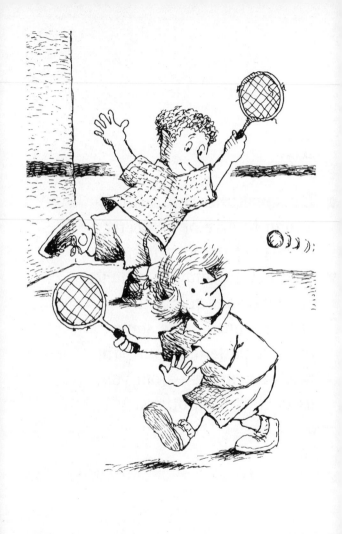

13.

It's sometimes difficult as
a man to give or to receive,
because of the masculine
tendency toward self-reliance.
Let your loss give you
permission to break some
of these patterns. Your pain
needs attention—from you,
as well as from others.

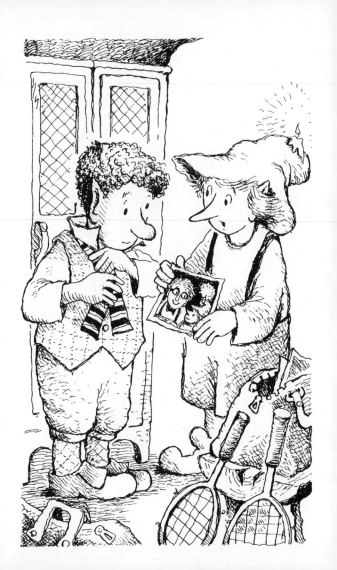

14.

If you're wary of "going public" with your grief, carefully select just one or two people in whom to confide. Start by sharing your story with another man: a friend, an uncle, your father, a brother or cousin.

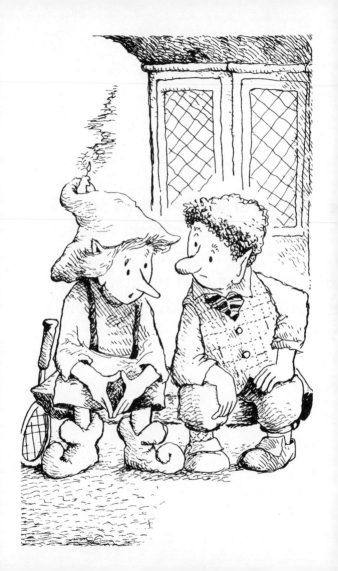

15.

If hugs or touching don't seem
comfortable, try a phone call
or a letter. You can express a
good deal of grief in these ways
without baring your entire soul.

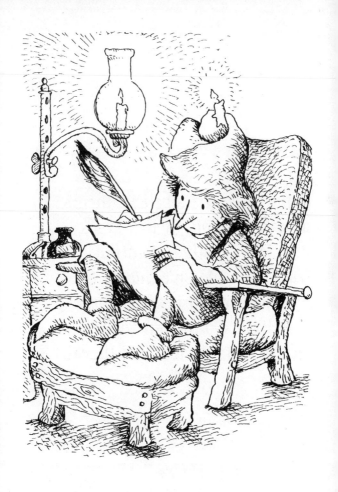

16.

Some researchers believe there's a male hormone which keeps men from easily generating tears. That doesn't change the fact that crying is well worth the effort. Go to your room and let the tears come when they're there.

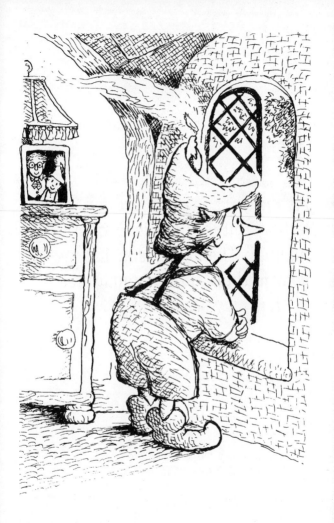

17.

As men, we need to feel our feelings rather than just to manfully "handle" them. Let your feelings surface, unnatural as that may seem.

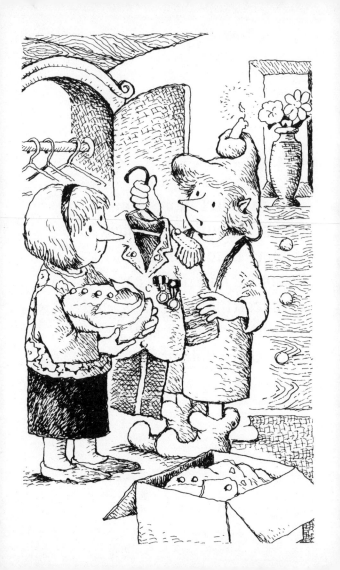

18.

Grief may feel more like confusion, guilt, numbness, or anger than sadness. Recognize and tackle each of these legitimate feelings, and you will be more likely to tackle the whole of it.

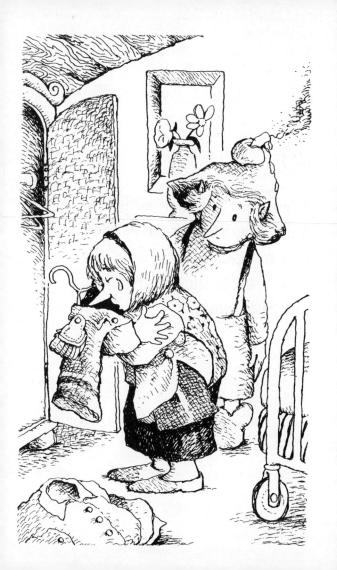

19.

Men especially can suffer the guilt of failing to fix everything and rescue everyone from this loss. Accept that your title is not Superman.

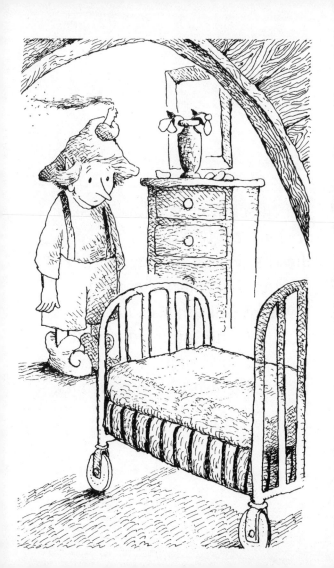

20.

When someone you love dies,
it can seem like the end of your
dreams. Worse, it may feel like
failure. Remember that your
loved one's death was not a
result of your failure, and that
God and love have the power to
restore the heart of your dreams.

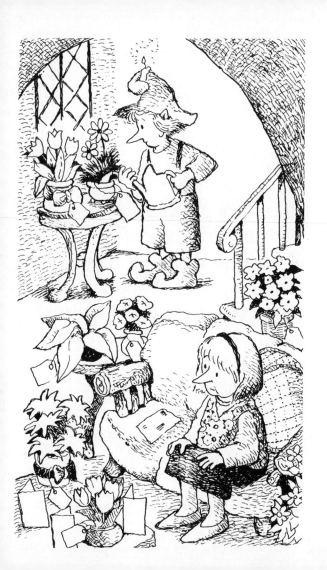

21.

When someone you love dies, you might experience feelings of relief along with feelings of deep sadness. These are not just "efficient, male feelings"—these are human feelings that are part of the normal grief process. Accept them.

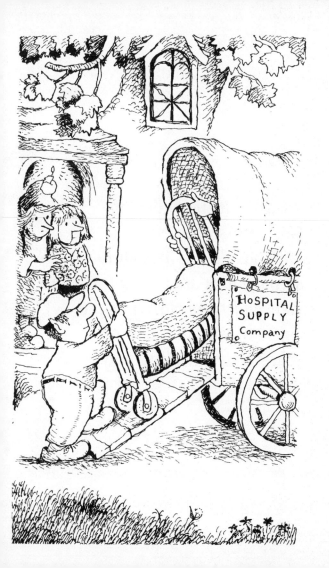

22.

Anger—at life, a doctor, God, yourself, or even the one who has died—frequently accompanies grief. Acknowledge your anger to yourself or the object of your anger in a constructive, healthy way.

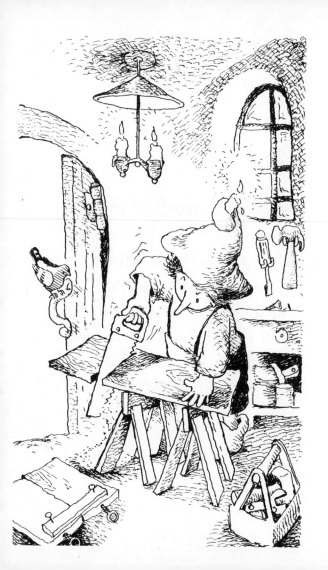

23.

Put anger to work for you—
not against you. Channel your
energies to help prevent others
from suffering the kind of
tragedy your loved one suffered.
Great comfort and healing can
come from this kind of work.

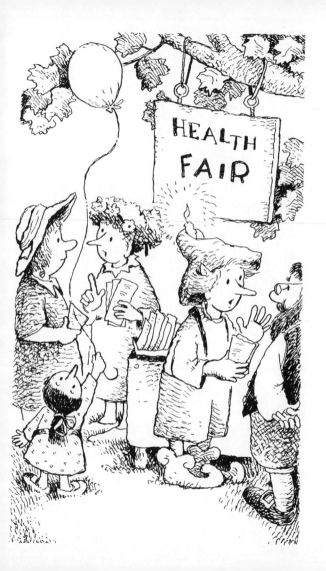

24.

Real men can get scared. It's normal to wonder and worry about what's next. Real courage means acknowledging fears— not denying they exist. Face your fears.

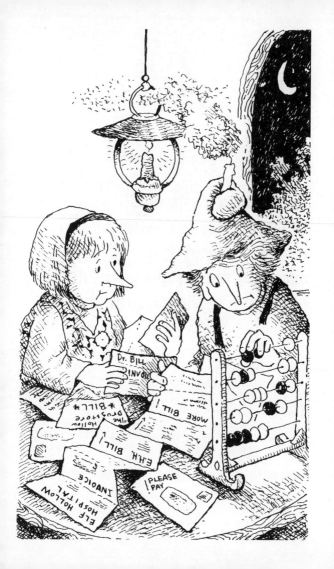

25.

Be courageous in small, measured steps. You don't have to do everything, all at once, full force, right away, all the way. Do the next thing.

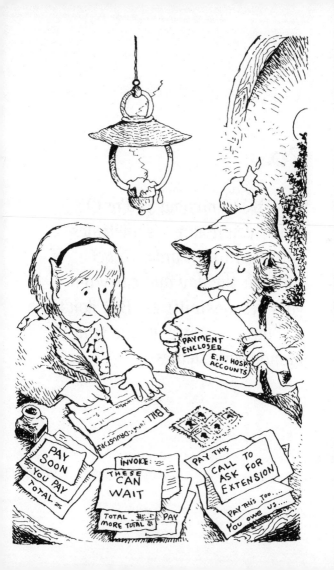

26.

It's OK to pretend you're OK when you're not—sometimes you need to, in order to get through the day and carry out your responsibilities. But don't put on a pretense all the time. Honor your sadness.

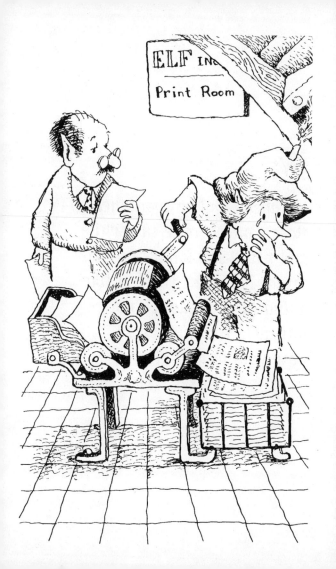

27.

Go ahead and be spontaneous—
"lose control" once in awhile
and really say what's on your
mind. Do what you feel like
doing (as long as it's not
hurtful). You know best
how you need to grieve.

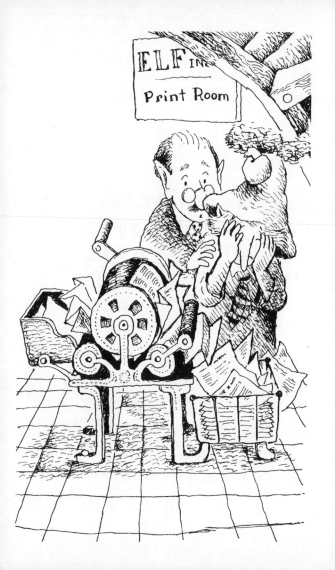

28.

Being very adept at doing things, you may feel especially frustrated that there is little or nothing you can do to help matters now. Sometimes action is overrated. Practice just being—by yourself, with God, or with a trusted friend. Being may come harder than doing, but it is necessary for balance.

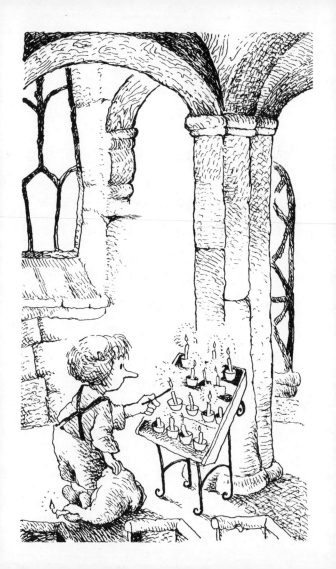

29.

Sitting quietly with your feelings may be the last thing you want to do as a man. Indeed, the hardest of all things to do is to do "nothing." Yet when you look quietly toward the doorway to your soul, you can enter a place of relief and peace.

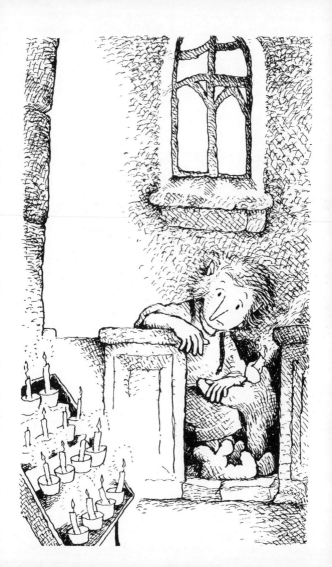

30.

If praying comes hard, recognize that your yelling or crying is itself prayer. It is surely what our loving God expects from us in the midst of pain.

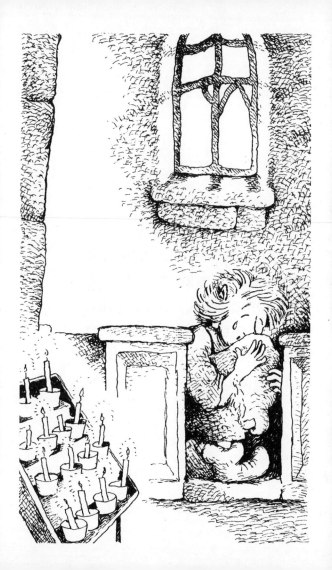

31.

Your family and intimate friends are most likely to give you the support and grief-space you need. But keep in mind that sometimes an "outsider," such as a therapist, minister, or counselor, can be a valuable sounding board.

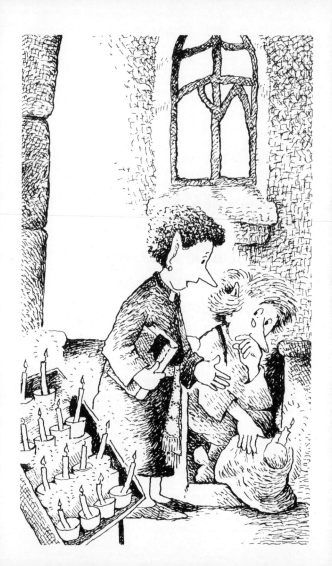

32.

Men don't like to leave "unfinished business." Take time to make amends, offer forgiveness, or express your feelings to help clear up leftover emotional business.

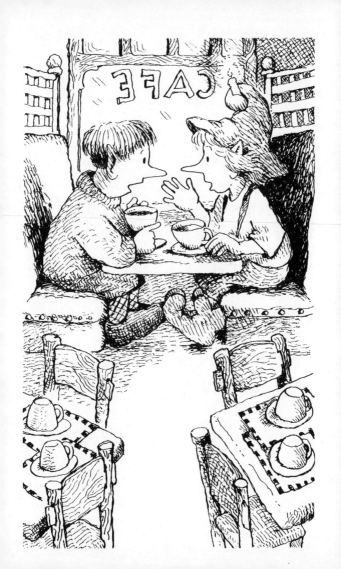

33.

If closeness and tenderness don't come naturally for you, you may need to sharpen your emotional "tools" to dig out these deeply suppressed parts of yourself. Start digging. The buried treasures you uncover will serve you well.

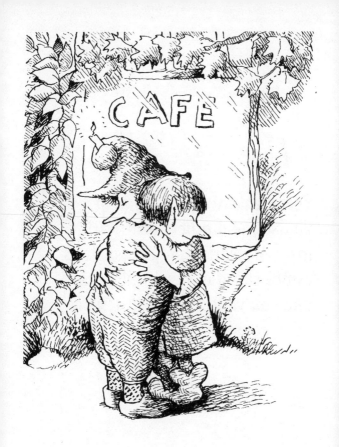

34.

Seek healthy rituals to help yourself and others deal with loss. A creative project, such as establishing a memorial to the one you've loved and lost, is a truly constructive action.

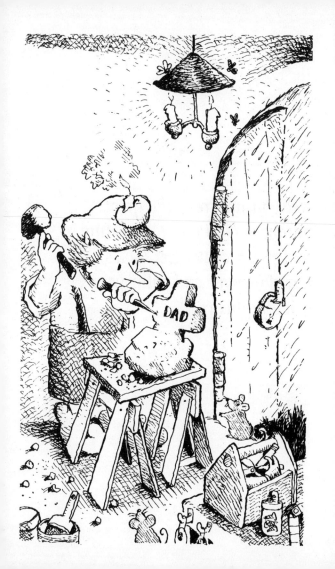

35.

Rely on nature—the great outdoors—to provide nurture and perspective. Let God's big sky cover and calm your grieving heart.

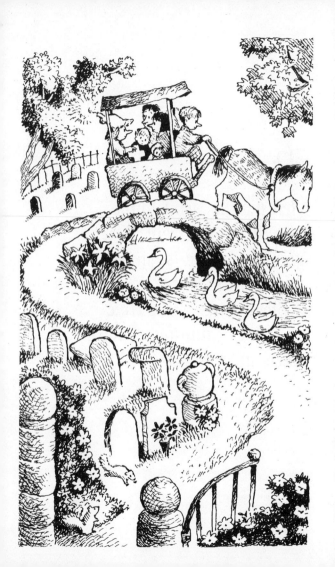

36.

Men tend to want to fix everything—quickly. But after loss, peace is gained only in little pieces. Lots of them. This is the time for small beginnings—with others at your side.

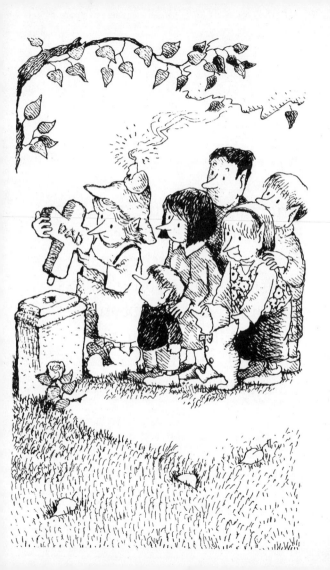

37.

Grief can become the "necessary wounding" that men need in order to see themselves more realistically: less powerful, less in control, and less robotic— but more human than ever imagined. Honor the transforming power of grief.

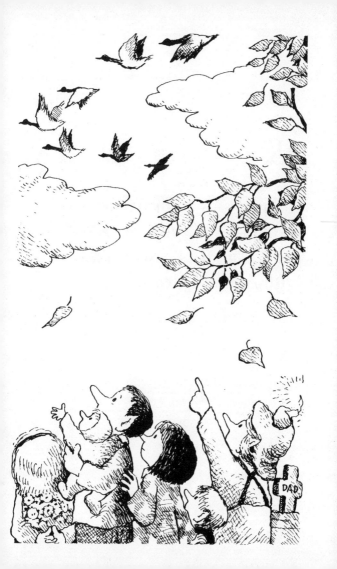

38.

For men—as with women—
there is a path from grief to
grace. And it is best walked
with Another. Reach out.

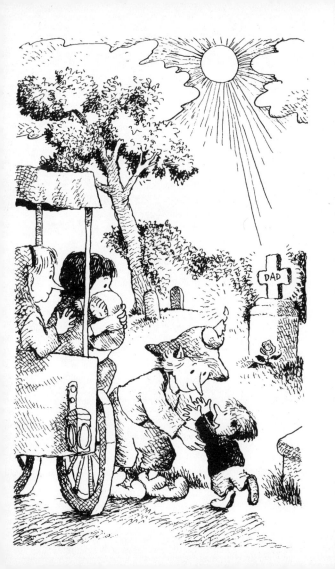

Linus Mundy is director of Publications at Abbey Press. Married and the father of three children, he has also written *Slow-down Therapy*, *Keep-life-simple Therapy* and *Everyday-courage Therapy* in the Elf-help Book series.

Illustrator for the Abbey Press Elf-help Books, **R.W. Alley** also illustrates and writes children's books. He lives in Barrington, Rhode Island, with his wife, daughter, and son.

The Story of the Abbey Press Elves

The engaging figures that populate the Abbey Press "elf-help" line of publications and products first appeared in 1987 on the pages of a small self-help book called *Be-good-to-yourself Therapy*. Shaped by the publishing staff's vision and defined in R.W. Alley's inventive illustrations, they lived out author Cherry Hartman's gentle, self-nurturing advice with charm, poignancy, and humor.

Reader response was so enthusiastic that more Elf-help Books were soon under way, a still-growing series that has inspired a line of related gift products.

The especially endearing character featured in the early books—sporting a cap with a mood-changing candle in its peak—has since been joined by a spirited female elf with flowers in her hair.

These two exuberant, sensitive, resourceful, kindhearted, lovable sprites, along with their lively elfin community, reveal what's truly important as they offer messages of joy and wonder, playfulness and co-creation, wholeness and serenity, the miracle of life and the mystery of God's love.

With wisdom and whimsy, these little creatures with long noses demonstrate the elf-help way to a rich and fulfilling life.

Elf-help Books

...adding "a little character" and a lot of help to self-help reading!

Grief Therapy for Men
#20141 $4.95   ISBN 0-87029-306-0

New Baby Therapy
#20140 $4.95   ISBN 0-87029-307-9

Living From Your Soul
#20146 $4.95   ISBN 0-87029-303-6

Teacher Therapy
#20145 $4.95   ISBN 0-87029-302-8

Be-good-to-your-family Therapy
#20154 $4.95   ISBN 0-87029-300-1

Stress Therapy
#20153 $4.95   ISBN 0-87029-301-X

Making-sense-out-of-suffering Therapy
#20156 $4.95   ISBN 0-87029-296-X

Get Well Therapy
#20157 $4.95   ISBN 0-87029-297-8

Anger Therapy
#20127 $4.95   ISBN 0-87029-292-7

Caregiver Therapy
#20164 $4.95   ISBN 0-87029-285-4

Self-esteem Therapy
#20165 $4.95   ISBN 0-87029-280-3

Take-charge-of-your-life Therapy
#20168 $4.95   ISBN 0-87029-271-4

Work Therapy
#20166 $4.95   ISBN 0-87029-276-5

Everyday-courage Therapy
#20167 $4.95   ISBN 0-87029-274-9

Peace Therapy
#20176 $4.95   ISBN 0-87029-273-0

Friendship Therapy
20174 $4.95   ISBN 0-87029-270-6

Christmas Therapy (color edition)
20175 $5.95   ISBN 0-87029-268-4

Grief Therapy
20178 $4.95   ISBN 0-87029-267-6

More Be-good-to-yourself Therapy
20180 $3.95   ISBN 0-87029-262-5

Happy Birthday Therapy
#20181 $4.95   ISBN 0-87029-260-9

Forgiveness Therapy
#20184 $4.95   ISBN 0-87029-258-7

Keep-life-simple Therapy
#20185 $4.95   ISBN 0-87029-257-9

Be-good-to-your-body Therapy
#20188 $4.95   ISBN 0-87029-255-2

Celebrate-your-womanhood Therapy
#20189 $4.95   ISBN 0-87029-254-4

Acceptance Therapy (color edition)
#20182 $5.95   ISBN 0-87029-259-5

Acceptance Therapy
#20190 $4.95   ISBN 0-87029-245-5

Keeping-up-your-spirits Therapy
#20195 $4.95   ISBN 0-87029-242-0

Play Therapy
#20200 $4.95   ISBN 0-87029-233-1

Slow-down Therapy
#20203 $4.95   ISBN 0-87029-229-3

One-day-at-a-time Therapy
#20204 $4.95   ISBN 0-87029-228-5

Prayer Therapy
#20206 $4.95   ISBN 0-87029-225-0

Be-good-to-your-marriage Therapy
#20205 $4.95   ISBN 0-87029-224-2

Be-good-to-yourself Therapy (hardcover)
#20196 $10.95   ISBN 0-87029-243-9

Be-good-to-yourself Therapy
#20255 $4.95   ISBN 0-87029-209-9

Available at your favorite bookstore or directly
from us at: One Caring Place, Abbey Press
Publications, St. Meinrad, IN 47577.
Or call 1-800-325-2511.